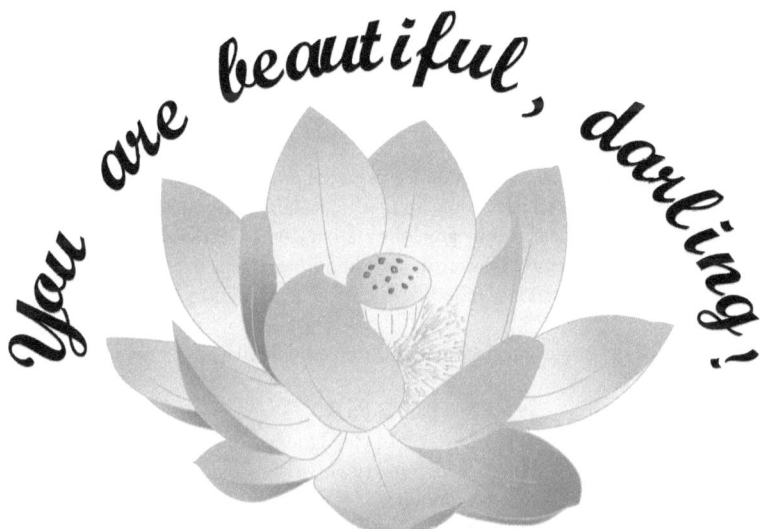

You are beautiful, darling!

A first-aid kit for stressed out women

Neli P. Georgieva

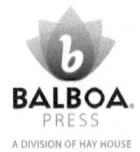

BALBOA.
PRESS
A DIVISION OF HAY HOUSE

Acknowledgements for images
Denor Media
Enroc Illustration

Balboa Press books may be ordered through booksellers or by contacting:

Balboa Press
A Division of Hay House
1663 Liberty Drive
Bloomington, IN 47403
www.balboapress.com
1 (877) 407-4847

Because of the dynamic nature of the Internet, any web addresses or links contained in this book may have changed since publication and may no longer be valid. The views expressed in this work are solely those of the author and do not necessarily reflect the views of the publisher, and the publisher hereby disclaims any responsibility for them.

The author of this book does not dispense medical advice or prescribe the use of any technique as a form of treatment for physical, emotional, or medical problems without the advice of a physician, either directly or indirectly. The intent of the author is only to offer information of a general nature to help you in your quest for emotional and spiritual well-being. In the event you use any of the information in this book for yourself, which is your constitutional right, the author and the publisher assume no responsibility for your actions.

Any people depicted in stock imagery provided by Thinkstock are models, and such images are being used for illustrative purposes only. Certain stock imagery © Thinkstock.

Print information available on the last page.

ISBN: 978-1-5043-4589-7 (sc)
ISBN: 978-1-5043-4590-3 (e)

Balboa Press rev. date: 1/19/2016

Table of Contents

Foreword

Hello darling,

You are the most important person on this planet. So, it is very important that you accept and love yourself.

I am here to help you.

Why am I writing this book?

In today's society, stress and burnout seem to be accepted as the norm. They are part of everyday life. We do not talk about them because these topics are not appropriate. If you happen to be affected, you feel ashamed because you are not as strong as you are supposed to be. So, you just think to yourself: "Pull yourself together and go on!" You pull yourself together once, you pull yourself together twice, and a couple of more times until you notice that this is no longer possible. So, you failed. You failed the expectations of your company, you failed the expectations of your family, you failed the expectations of your friends, and you failed the expectations of yourself.

You are supposed to give. You are supposed to give to your company in the form of overtime hours and superior performance. You are supposed to give time and energy to relatives because if you don't, you are seen as selfish and uncaring. You are supposed to give, give, give…

Now, let's be honest. If this was all how it was supposed to be, why have you reached this point? Are you close to burnout? Are you depressed? Are you feeling hopeless and unsure what to do with your life?

If you have answered, "Yes" to any of these questions, stop reading. Go and look at yourself in the mirror. Do you feel like crying? It's ok to cry because now we want to focus on YOU.

YOU are the most important person on the planet. You deserve to be happy, to feel good and to love yourself. Forget about what everyone else is saying.

So first, we need to take care of you. Put that smile back on your face – yes, you deserve to smile! You deserve to feel beautiful.

My motivation for writing is very simple: I have seen too many people encounter burnout. The worst part is, it has become accepted as the norm. During one of my projects, there was a French woman who I often talked to on the phone. One day, this woman told me there was too much pressure, and the company had too many expectations. The deadlines were not realistic, the work was piling up, and the staff was halved. She explained that she needed to go because she had to pick up her small daughter from kindergarten. Two days later, this woman ended up in a psychiatric hospital. She could not handle the work pressure.

I quit the project, and I felt responsible for what had happened to her.

Later on, I ended up working on a new project in which out of ten people in the particular team, five had "collapsed" because of stress related to work. Indeed, if you read job advertisements, you see the description "flexible, multitasking, and resilient" quite often. Firms are nowadays frequently looking for people who can handle a fast pace, and maybe YOU don't belong there. I will encourage you to look honestly at whether your workplace is giving you what you need for your personal well-being, but more of that later. First, let's make you happy and healthy again.

Since this book is dedicated to us, WOMEN, we will also look into how stress and burnout affect your femininity and self-confidence, and what you can do to get these back.

I hope that this small booklet, written in an authentic everyday language, will help you get back to your best.

We first want you to be HAPPY and HEALTHY before you make any other decisions to re-evaluate YOUR life.

1. Stress and burnout

"Burnout is nature's way of telling you, you've been going through the motions, your soul has departed; you're a zombie, a member of the walking dead, a sleepwalker. False optimism is like administrating stimulants to an exhausted nervous system."

-Sam Keen-

Burnout incidences rise exponentially. These statistics have been proven scientifically. Here are some interesting facts based on statistics in Germany:

- In 2011, 59.2 million disability days were due to mental illness in Germany. That is an increase of more than 80 percent in the last 15 years.
- Up to 13 million people in Germany are affected by burnout (estimates of health professionals and health insurance agencies). The German population is about 82 million people.
- Nearly ten million days were spent on sick leave because of burnout symptoms in 2010. In other words, around 40,000 workers were missing throughout the year in the office because they suffered from burnout.

- Twenty percent of all workers experience burnout-similar symptoms, which means that every fifth person is affected.
- A burnout causes on average 30.4 sick days per year, as shown by studies of the World Health Organization (WHO).
- One in five workers suffers from health consequences of stress - from insomnia to heart attack.
- Every third employed person works at the limit and feels strongly depleted.
- 41 percent of all inflows into pension for reduced earning capacity were due to mental disorders.
- Mental stress is therefore now the number one cause of early retirement. The average age was 48.3 years.

Many people suffering from burnout are between 30 and 45 years old. These are people who are ambitious and results-driven. They are perfectionists. They do not like to fail expectations, either their own or the expectations of the people around them. It is normally people who never believed that burnout could become their problem. They noticed the stress, they noticed tension, but they ignored their own body's signals: giving up or slowing down is associated with failure.

Women who try to juggle job and family life with kids are particularly susceptible to burnout when they want to live up to all the expectations put on them: be a perfect mother, be good at your job, have a 90-60-90 body, be a great wife... (fill in the dots). These women try to fulfill all expectations put on them and be great at each different area.

I found a nice quote from *Psychology Today* that I would like to share with you:

> *"The seeds of burnout get planted as early as high school.*
> *High-achieving girls and boys get the message early on*

that if they are to get into a top school and succeed in life, they must excel in every area – grades, friendships, volunteering, extracurricular activities and more.

Messages about self-care and the importance of recovery aren't always sent as strongly as messages about achievement and success, and that has implications for how women eventually work, live, and parent."[1]

So, when you can't get out of bed because of depression and/or burnout, when you can't bear the pressure of all this: then you are a BIG FAILURE. This is how we think. Do you see the vicious cycle here?

I have come to believe that we need to learn to follow a healthy rhythm. A rhythm that does not lead to stress and back pain. But first we need to learn what is good for us and for our bodies. And then follow through – both in our work and private lives. You still can't say "no" to your boss who wants you to stay in the office until 10 p.m.? Or accept behaviours from your egocentric friends that you do not agree with just to keep up the peace? This is why you are reading this book.

You would have to develop a habit of setting healthy boundaries and putting your own needs first. You can only be respected and appreciated by others if you respect and appreciate yourself first. And if you still do not get the respect that you deserve in your current environment, you would need the courage to move on and surround yourself with people who really appreciate you.

---

[1] "Why Some Women Are Burning Out in Their 20's and 30's." Psychology Today. Web. 26 Aug. 2015.

Once you find yourself in the company of supportive friends and a team-oriented company culture, you can feel much better about yourself. It is just as easy to feel good about ourselves in the company of supporting and uplifting people as it is to feel bad about ourselves if we are constantly put down and criticized, or have to deal with unrealistic expectations.

2. It's *ME* time

Women react in a different way to stress than men. If a woman does not have time to take care of herself, her perception of being feminine suffers which leads to lower self-esteem. In addition, there is evidence that high levels of stress speed up the aging process.

Does stress make you feel ugly?

I would not be surprised if you say yes. Stress has a direct impact on beauty. As Robert Tornambe wrote in an article on Huffington Post:

> *"Stress that is not controlled most certainly affects the body's physical characteristics or beauty. It affects skin, hair, fingernails, digestion and sleep patterns. Stress-induced conditions include hair loss, heart disease, obesity, obsessive-compulsive disorder, sexual dysfunction, tooth and gum disease and ulcers or indigestion."*[2]

On top of this, a lot of women tend to exaggerate their problems and be extremely harsh on themselves. In stressful situations, this

---

[2] Tornambe, M.D. "Does Stress Make You Ugly?" *The Huffington Post.* TheHuffingtonPost.com. Web. 26 Aug. 2015.

could have the effect of making you even more stressed out without you even realizing it.

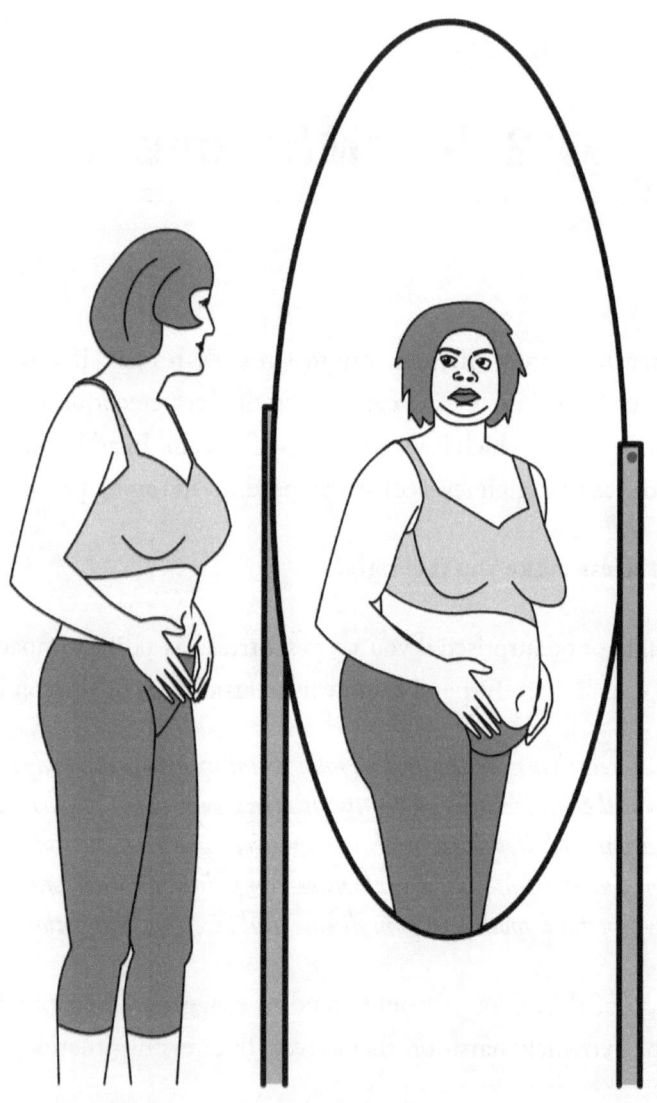

Once you are able to relax and connect to your inner self, you start to feel beautiful again and emerge in your feminine energy. Say out loud to yourself a couple of times: "You are beautiful, darling!" Experience how these words resonate within you. Be patient with yourself and do something nice to cherish your presence in the world every day.

2.1. Relaxation, meditation, awareness, resilience

Relaxation

First of all, it is important to create time and space for relaxation. Take a couple of days only for yourself. Do something that you enjoy – drawing, dancing, singing are some examples of such activities. Get a massage. Go for a manicure and pedicure or get a haircut. Gift yourself a facial. I personally find swimming and sauna very relaxing. Take the time to slide into the day and do whatever you feel like doing.

If you have the urge to go back to your "TO DO" list, don't. This is a side result of your perfectionism; the mind finds it difficult to be confronted with emptiness and lack of purpose. But it is exactly this emptiness that is necessary for you to learn to feel and understand your body and your own needs. I found a wonderful quote from Thich Nhat Hanh which I would like to share with you: **"The seed of suffering in you may be strong, but don't wait until you have no more suffering before allowing yourself to be happy."**[3]

Next, go out and talk to people. It is important that you surround yourself with positive people and do not keep your woes to yourself.

---

[3] "Thich-nhat-hanh-quotes." - Mystical Earth Adventures™. Web. 26 Aug. 2015.

Talk to people who can listen without judging. If you do not have any friends and feel lonely, look up some gatherings in your city (Meet-up, Spontacts, Internations). It is possible that you would have to attend a couple of these organized events before you meet people who have similar interests. Do not be afraid to try out new events and stay open for what presents itself.

However, be careful not to end up in the company of manipulative people who would use your openness and vulnerability. If in doubt, stop contact with these individuals until you feel better and ready to make a decision about the particular situation. There are always enough other people to meet and talk to.

Do the things which you have postponed and which you have always wanted to try. Don't take yourself seriously. Talk to people who you would normally not talk to. Take the time to just *BE*: ENJOY nature, ENJOY the sun and the company of the most important person on the planet - YOU.

Meditation

Meditation is helpful to quieten the mind and let go of all the whys and hows and guilt feelings you have about not measuring up to your own expectations and the expectations of people around you.

Be easy on yourself. It is important that you are here, alive and that you have a chance to re-evaluate your life. Think of all the people with heart attacks who lead a similar lifestyle and for whom there is no coming back, no second chance. This should, by the way, also bring you to the question: "What am I doing with my life?" Which is in itself a very confusing question and you do not have to answer it right away. First take the time to feel healthy and happy again.

Do you still feel guilty? Go out and look at the sun. The sun is just shining at you and does not want anything in return. It is so easy to forget these feelings of guilt and shame when basking under sunlight. So, if you live in a warm country, pack your bathing stuff and go sit somewhere in the outdoors.

Back to the subject of meditation. When you start searching for spirituality and the meaning of life, or at least trying to make sense of your current situation, you will be confronted with a lot of offers. Different books, different schools, different lines of thought offer you "spiritual enlightenment" if you sign up for their course. If you are not sure, it is better to be careful and to request further information. You are probably weaker than you normally are, so it is extremely important to choose your influencers at this moment wisely. Stay away from anything weird or stuff that you do not trust.

Of the different courses and meditation workshops I tried, I would say that Zen is very nice. In most big cities, there are Zen meditation centres that offer meditations for free or for a small donation. Again, if anyone is trying to put you under pressure to sign up for a course or go to an event – this might not be the right one for you. You can ask what the meditation teacher thinks about other schools or lines of thought. If he or she downplays the others or tells you this is the only truth, I would advise you to not go to this place again.

Zen meditation helps you focus on your breathing which has a calming effect on your mind. Learning to breathe deeply will help you for the next step in the journey: awareness and self-observance.

You can try some meditation at home. You can start with a ten-minute daily breathing meditation and slowly increase the amount of time you spend. It is important that you build the meditation practice into your daily routine and be patient with yourself.

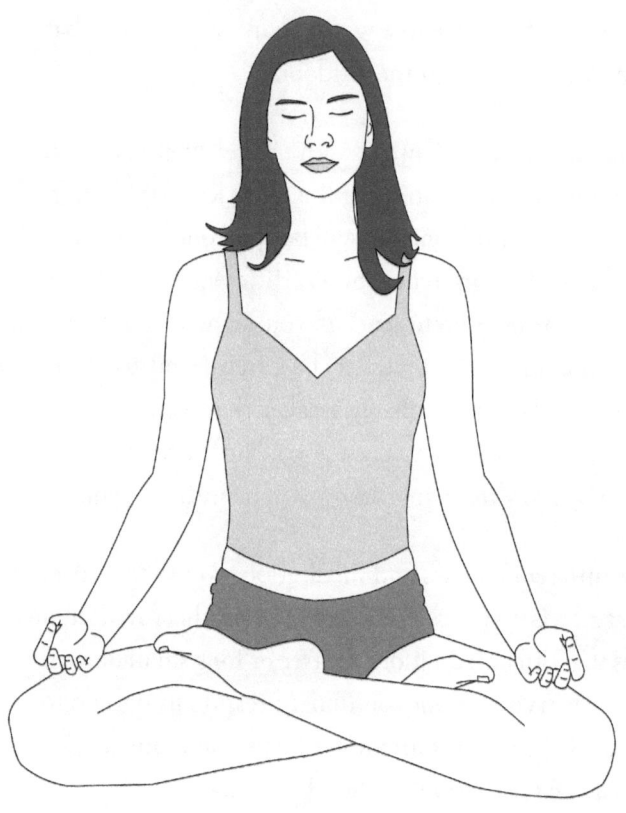

In order to meditate, find a comfortable sitting position. You can either sit on the floor with crossed legs as the woman in the picture above or sit on a chair. If you sit on a chair, do not cross your legs and have the feet touching the floor. You can put the hands either on your crotch or resting on your thighs as illustrated above. Turn the palms of the hands towards the ceiling. The thumb and index fingers touch, the other fingers are relaxed.

With the practice of meditation, you learn to observe your own thoughts and accept them as they come without identifying yourself with them. This is a marvellous process in helping you to change your thought patterns. Of course, the first step to changing your thought patterns is recognizing them.

Many healers and alternative medicine practitioners make an hour of meditation a daily exercise. Some split this time in chunks of 15-20 minute meditation sessions after waking up, at lunch and before going to bed. During the meditation practice, you can connect with your inner guidance and explore the source of peace and quietness coming from within yourself.

Speaking meta sentences for yourself and others is a very good enhancement to your meditation practice. Speaking or chanting *meta* sentences can be done at home and requires only a couple of minutes of your time. And it feels great. So, here is how it goes: "May I be happy. May I be healthy. May I be safe. May I have an easy-going and untroubled life!" Or, "May you be happy. May you be healthy. May you be safe. May you have an easy-going and untroubled life!" Or, "May everyone be happy. May everyone be healthy. May everyone be safe. May everyone have an easy-going and untroubled life!"

Spirituality is a personal choice. I would encourage you to try the exercises above – it is up to you what you choose to believe in. Everyone believes in something.

Awareness

Gaining awareness is a process and requires you to be patient.

Awareness is important so that you are able to recognize your own thought and stress patterns. So, if you recognize any of these: wanting to do many things at the same time, being polite and having difficulty saying no, needing to do something just to stay busy... Fill in the blanks: we will have a lot of work to do ☺

Meditation will help you to become more aware of your thought patterns and habits. The idea is that you first need to observe yourself in order to realise your thought and behaviour patterns. Once you do, you can consciously decide to change them. In the process, be nice to yourself and take your spiritual journey at a pace that you are comfortable with.

For example, I observed that I am a perfectionist and that I put myself under pressure sometimes without a reason. Now that I am aware of this, I can observe myself and change my behaviour whenever I fall into this pattern.

Developing awareness is a process. If you have time, set aside one to two hours each day only for yourself to develop your inner strength and clarity. You can decide which form of activity is right for you to support your self-discovery. Some examples of such activities are: Yoga, Meditation, Qi Gong and Tai Chi. You might decide that you would prefer a walk in nature so that you learn to enjoy your own company. A combination of different activities is excellent. The goal is for you to learn to do what is right for YOU and to trust your own judgement. You can recognize what is right for you when you have a feeling of lightness and happiness. It is ok to try out different activities until you find your own mix.

If you sometimes feel depressed again, remind yourself why you are taking this journey. It might be easy to stop doing the exploration exercises and fall back into your old patterns. You can sit at home and feel sorry for yourself all you want, but this will not change your life. You have the power to change your life, by changing the way you think and act at this present moment.

When you practice awareness, you will be able to notice in a timely manner when too much is going on and when to take care of yourself before getting stressed.

Resilience

Resilience is the ability to deal with changes and challenges. The root of the word comes from Latin and means "bouncing back" or "ricochet". With respect to stress, resilience is the ability to stay in control of the situation and react appropriately, while at the same time taking care of yourself. If the external events threaten to become too much of a challenge, a resilient person will notice this, take care of her own needs and communicate appropriate boundaries.

If you are resilient, your immune system functions correctly and it is easy for you to come back to a relaxed state of mind.

The discussion of resilience with respect to getting yourself out of a depression or burn-out is important. Building resilience can help you switch your perspective and see the positive sides of your situation. It will help you get out of the situation with more knowledge about yourself and what you want from your life.

A positive outlook towards life is resulting from the development of resilience and it will help you to see your situation from a different angle. In every situation, there is something positive and it is up to us to discover the positive aspects. With the focus in "Here and Now", we avoid falling pray to hope and pity. The strength lies within us in order to apply the "LVL" principle: Love it, Change it or Leave it. Only in the "Here and Now" it is possible to make decisions. As Thich Nhat Hanh puts it: *"People usually consider walking on water or in thin air a miracle. But I think the real miracle is not to walk either on water or in thin air, but to walk on earth."*[4]

So, if you have recently experienced stress or burnout, make a resolution NOW to learn how to take care of yourself and change your habits so that you start living a balanced life.

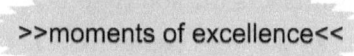

The balance model

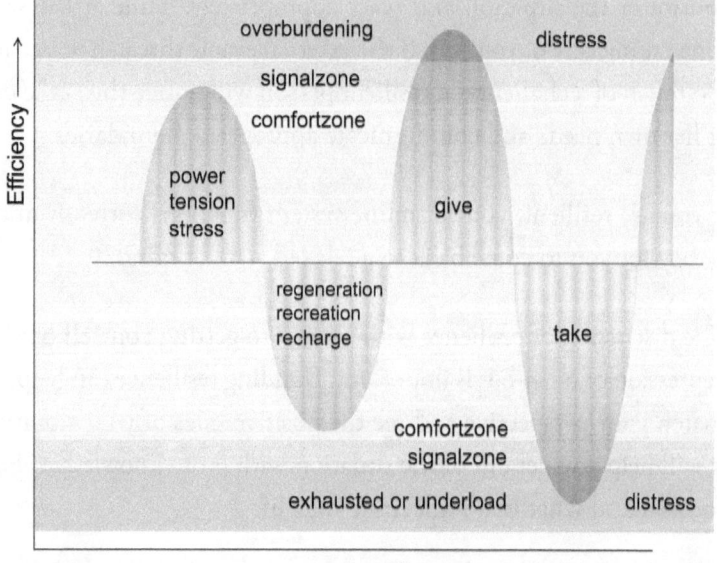

---

[4] "Thich-nhat-hanh-quotes." - Mystical Earth Adventures™. Web. 26 Aug. 2015.

In order to live in balance, you have to alter between phases of performance and phases of rest. In the image above, the so called "balance model", the middle part of the model indicates your comfort zone. If you spend too much time in "action" mode without having a proper rest phase, you run the danger of overstraining yourself and depleting your "batteries". It will take you a longer time to recharge and be able to perform at your normal level.

Aim to bring work, health, spirit and body in harmony – which is no easy task, but totally worth it.

2.2. Smile and enjoy life

No matter what your external circumstances happen to be, you can still smile and enjoy the moment. Happiness is a state and does not need to be tied to material positions or certain people in your life. If you want to be happy ... just allow yourself to be happy. You will see that this is much easier than you thought, and once you get used to this feeling of happiness, you will want to invite it into your life more and more often.

When you are happy, other people notice your state and react to it. You might be greeted by strangers on the street, or you might experience random people being extremely nice to you.

Remember – you carry this happiness in you – and are not dependent on the external circumstances to give it to yourself. When you reach this level of self-sufficient happiness, the external circumstances would start changing as well.

In Buddhism, this state of happiness is often described as a change of perception. If you are not dependent on your external circumstances, you are free. Stress is caused by not accepting the circumstances and wanting to be somewhere else. In the moment in which you accept the circumstances, you can act to change them. That is why there are so many writings about the power of NOW. Now is the only moment you can influence – you cannot change the past, so you might as well make peace with it. You do not own the future, so why focus so much on it? Even the best laid plans can turn out differently to the way you expected them to. So, go through life smiling – enjoying the present – which is the biggest PRESENT that you can give to yourself.

3. Stress revisited

A lot of the stress in our lives is self-created. This is why it is important to observe our patterns.

"The day has only 24 hours, and if these are not enough, I will also work at night." is a typical thinking pattern of ambitious and driven people.

A person who is under stress all the time will soon experience burnout. The high levels of activity get in the way of effective thinking. Even if you experience stress due to outside circumstances, you should still have time to take care of yourself and your personal needs.

This is YOUR life and it is therefore important that YOU consistently contemplate about what YOU expect from life, what is important to YOU and what YOU want to achieve.

It is YOUR responsibility to occasionally devote all your attention to the most important person in the world – YOU. Quality of life consists in finding the balance between career and private life and still having enough time for personal development. Dedicating too much time to your career and ignoring the other areas of your life leads in the long run to depressions and unhappiness. You do not have to take care of everything right away (multitasking), even if the tasks seem very interesting.

Each of us have a different mental set-up that activates stress. It is therefore good to keep a track record of your "stress patterns" and how you react in these types of situations. Once you recognize your pattern, you can choose to replace it with a new behaviour.

For example, these are some typical patterns and reactions:

Example 1:

External event: Someone wants something from you.

Typical pattern of reaction: You feel triggered. You feel like you have to react right away.

New pattern of reaction: Breathe deeply 5-10 times and ask yourself when you actually need to react. Put this date and time in your calendar.

Example 2:

External event: There is too much happening at the same time.

Typical pattern of reaction: Panic. The body tenses up. You feel like you will not be able to cope with all the tasks and demands placed on you.

New pattern of reaction: Take a break on purpose. Do things slower on purpose. Choose priorities. Learn to say "no".

Note: If you stop and think about your priorities, you will feel in control of the situation.

You can start making your "stress diary" and write down your observations before going to bed. Try out new patterns of behaviour during the day and check your progress in the evening.

You have to be patient with yourself and reward yourself for your progress. Change takes time.

In addition, you can reduce stress in your everyday life by trying some of these activities:

- Deep breathing (Focus on your breath for at least ten inhales and exhales.)
- Bringing yourself in motion:
  - do the Qi Gong exercise shown below
  - go up and down the stairs a couple of times

Observe how you feel after each activity.[5]

Qi Gong exercise

Qi Gong is an ancient Chinese form of exercise which involves the repetition of slow movements in order to help raise body awareness. Practicing Qi Gong has numerous health benefits:

"Many physical problems are at least partially due to, or aggravated by, mental or emotional stress, so the importance of the inner tranquility developed through chi gung cannot be overestimated. The practice of qigong helps manage the stress, anger, depression, morbid thoughts, and general confusion that prey on your mind when your chi is not regulated and balanced."[6]

---

[5] These exercises and activities have been shared by Carsten Stepan. For more information and contact, see references at the end of the book

[6] "What Is Qigong?" *Energy Arts*. Web. 27 Aug. 2015.

There is one particular Qi Gong exercise which can be done anywhere when you need to release stress and balance yourself. Stay in an upright position, with knees slightly bent. Bring your hands forward in front of your stomach around the area of the solar plexus, as shown in the image below.

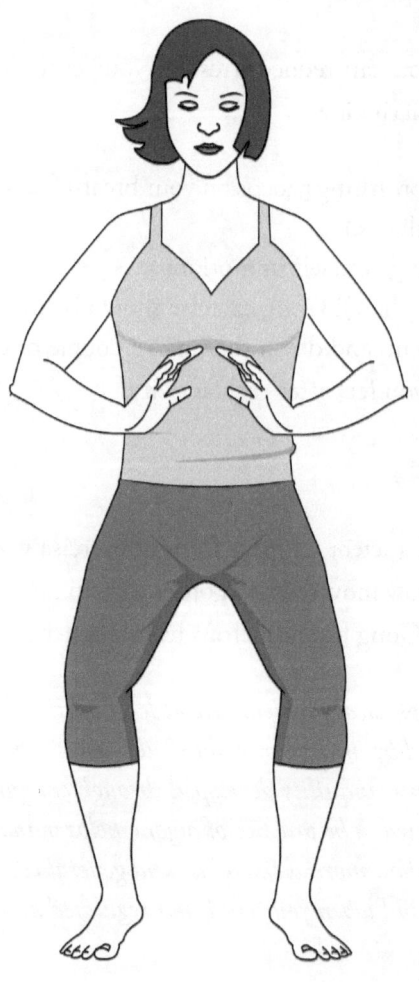

Imagine that you are holding a ball. Slowly move your hands up to the level of your neck and repeat to yourself: "I am calming my breathing" (see image on the next page).

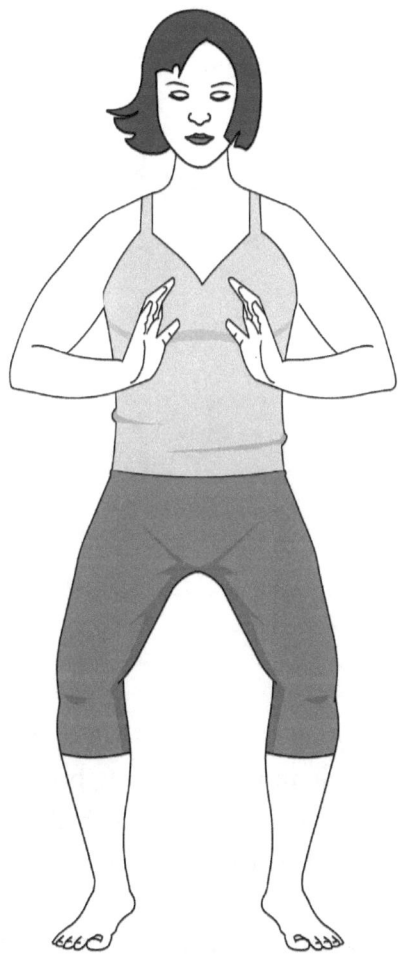

Then slowly move your hands down to the area of your stomach and repeat to yourself: "I am calming my mind."

Let me reiterate that coming to peace is totally worth the effort. A peaceful person radiates strength and sovereignty and conveys a feeling of security. This is so because contrary to most people who live a hectic and busy life, this person gives the impression of having control.

Do you want to be this person?

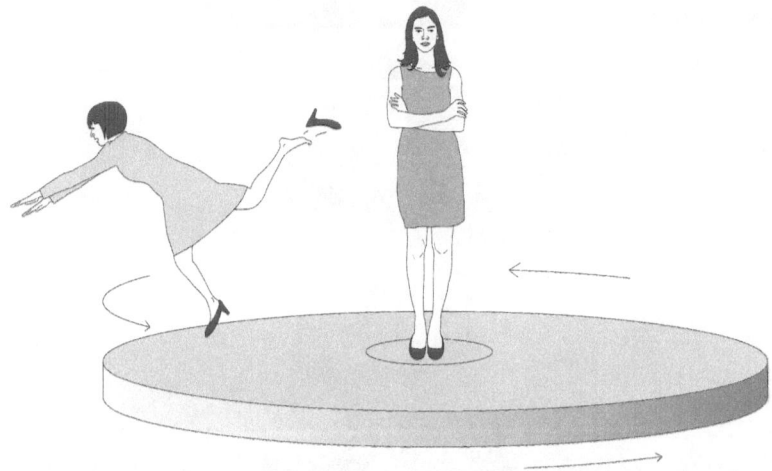

Centering

The activities happening in our lives seem to be important, hectic and urgent. We live at an ever-increasing pace. This causes stress because we do not know how to deal with all of the expectations thrown at us (juggling between job, family, gym, etc.)

More and more people have a yearning to be centred. To be centred means to remain calm even if external circumstances become crazy. I found this very nice definition of being centred which I would like to share with you:

"However, it is more difficult to "be centred" when things are happening in this instant that we would rather not be experiencing. [...]Being

centred means to be balanced in this instant one hundred percent, taking in information without clouding it with expectations or fear. Just taking in information and making creative, intuitive decisions informed by our "CENTER," our true intent, our original self.[7]

It is indeed an art to learn to be centred and at the same time, participate in your daily activities.

As Carsten Stepan shared in a workshop on stress management, remaining calm even if the external circumstances become "stormy" becomes easier with practice.

A good visual explanation for this balance between being centred and still taking part in your everyday life can be the Yin and Yang symbol which also explains the resolution of duality. In this symbol, you can see that the Yin is part of the Yang and the Yang is part of the Yin.

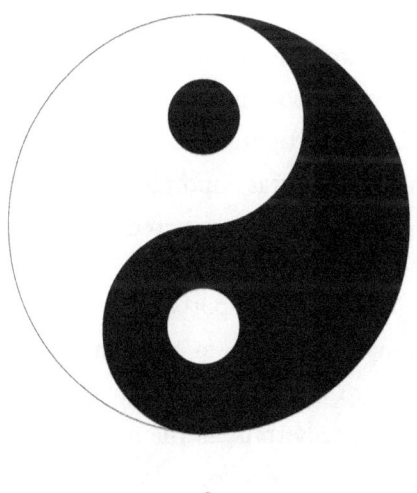

☺

---

[7] "What Does It Mean To Be Centered?" *What Does It Mean To Be Centered?* Web. 27 Aug. 2015.
https://www.jiyushinkai.org/centered.html

3.1. Fitness exercises that support you for your office job

Sport and relaxation are very important for patients suffering from burnout.

You do not have to wait to get burnout syndromes in order to take care of yourself. In the following pages, I will introduce you to a simple training plan to support you if you have an office job. Human beings are made to move, jump and run, so sitting around all day long lets our muscles degrade, which causes pain and many other problems. The back muscles should be moved and trained in order to regain their full functionality.

I have suffered from back and shoulder pain myself for quite a while now, so it was bliss to discover how simple the solution could be.

The idea behind the training is that most office jobs require us to sit for many hours in a row, so it is important to create endurance and resistance by training the right muscle groups: back, shoulders, and neck. During the training, it is important to develop body awareness of these muscle groups and how they move.

While we are often told to do sports, we often do not do the right training. For example, I was told to go swimming for my back pain. Swimming is great to get in shape and to keep a cardio workout, but it does not necessarily train all the muscle groups that we have to awake from being immobile for so long.

The back needs to be moved in all three directions: bend, stretch, and rotate. There are over 100 muscles in the back and they need to be trained regularly in order to function. When you understand what you are doing with each exercise, it is much easier to visualize the effect of the exercise on your body. With this awareness, you can focus on your training 100% in order to achieve the best results.

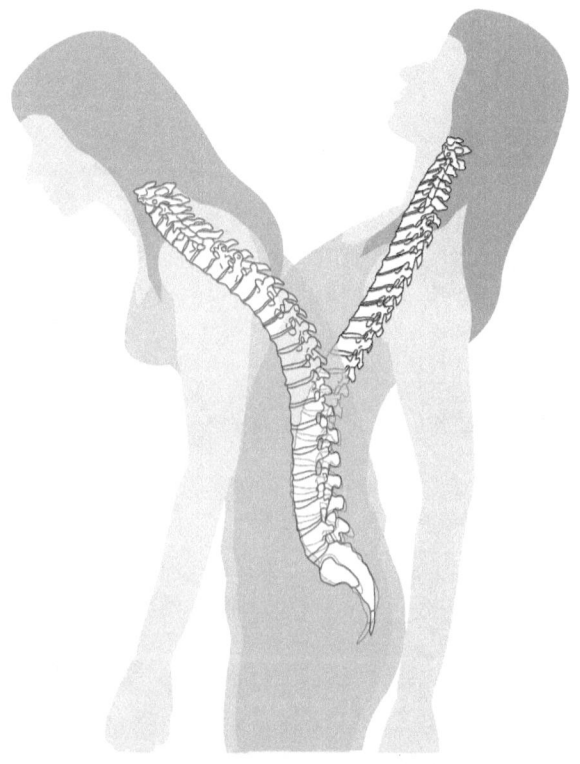

In addition, I would recommend you to do the so called "spinal massage" every two hours. You can set an alarm clock to remind yourself to get up and do these simple stretches at regular time intervals. It takes only about two minutes and it feels great.

Repeat each exercise 15-20 times.

Exercise 1:

Put two fingers on your chest, two fingers on your stomach to use as references (see images below). Then follow the pattern: chest in, chest out.

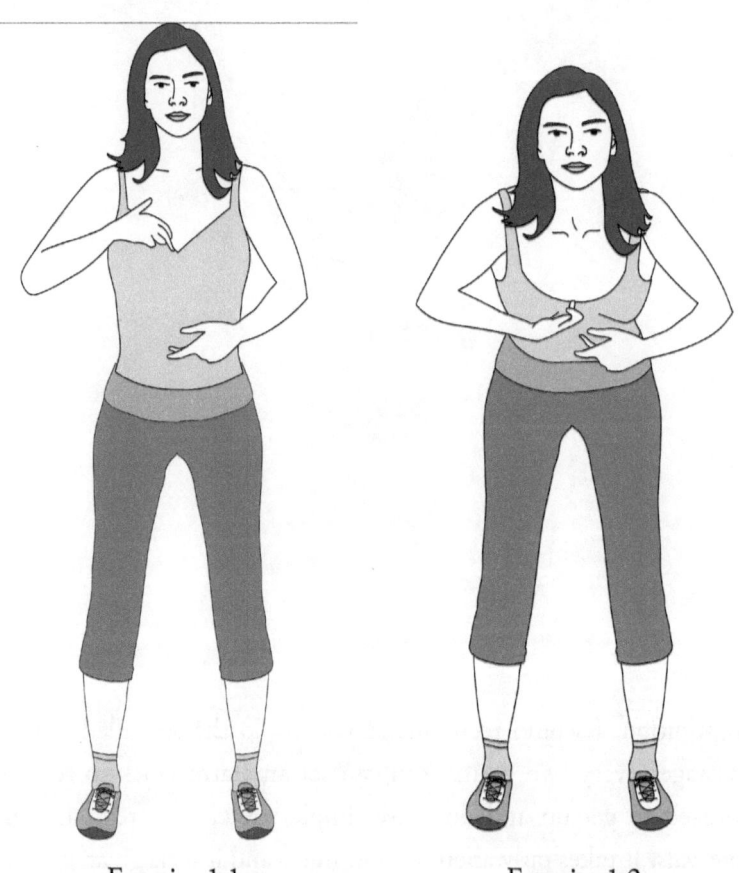

Exercise 1-1   Exercise 1-2

Exercise 2:

Bend to the floor and then stretch. For this exercise, it is important that the head is also included in the complete motion.

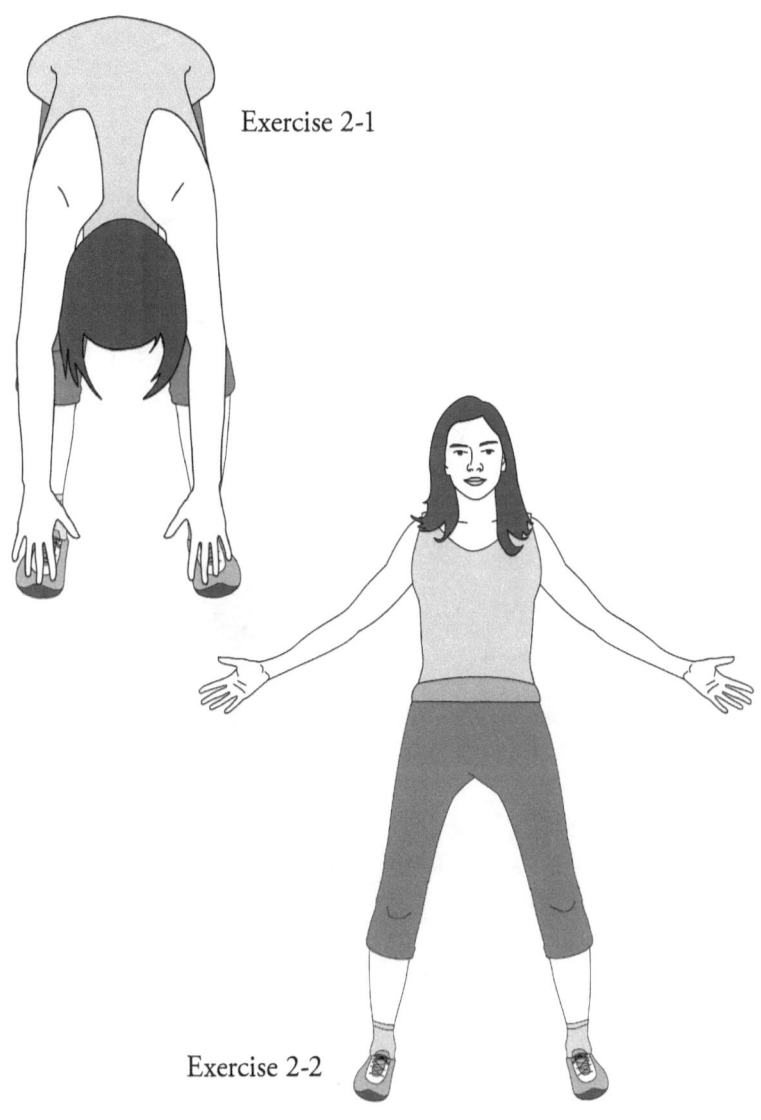

Exercise 2-1

Exercise 2-2

Exercise 3:

Bend to the right. Here it is important that the thighs do not move and that the movement is coming only from the spine.

Repeat the same exercise to the left.

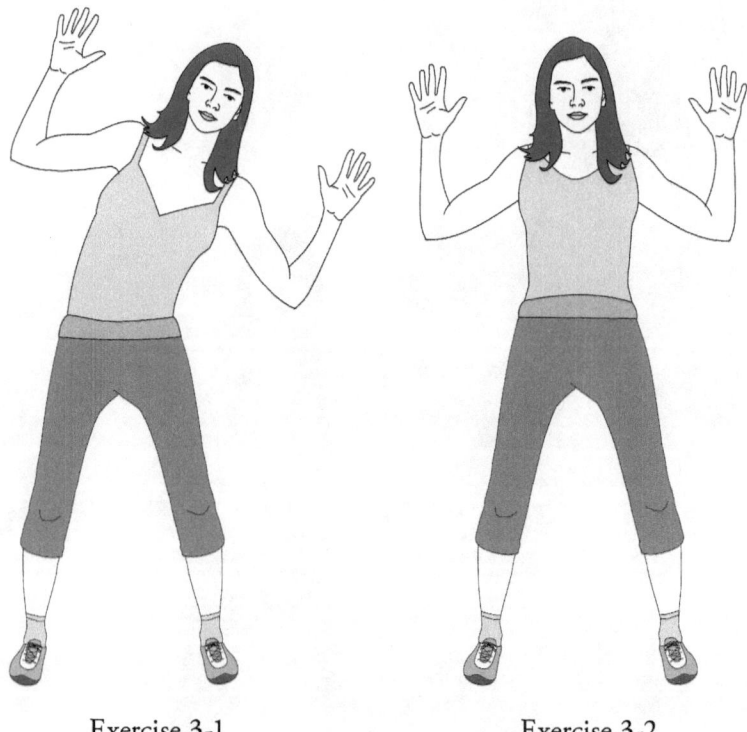

Exercise 3-1   Exercise 3-2

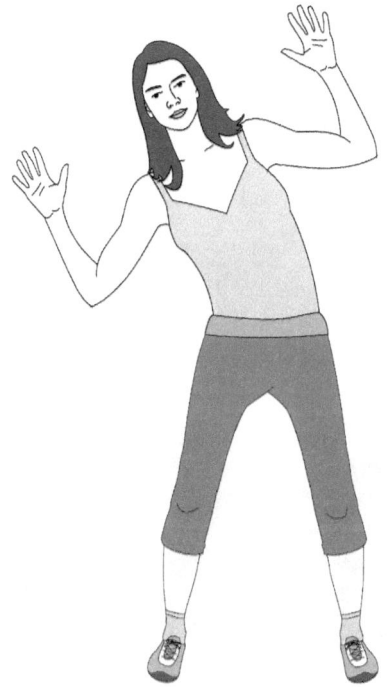

Exercise 3-3

Exercise 4:

Turn (rotate) to the back. Here, it is again important that the thighs do not move (see images below).

Repeat in both directions.

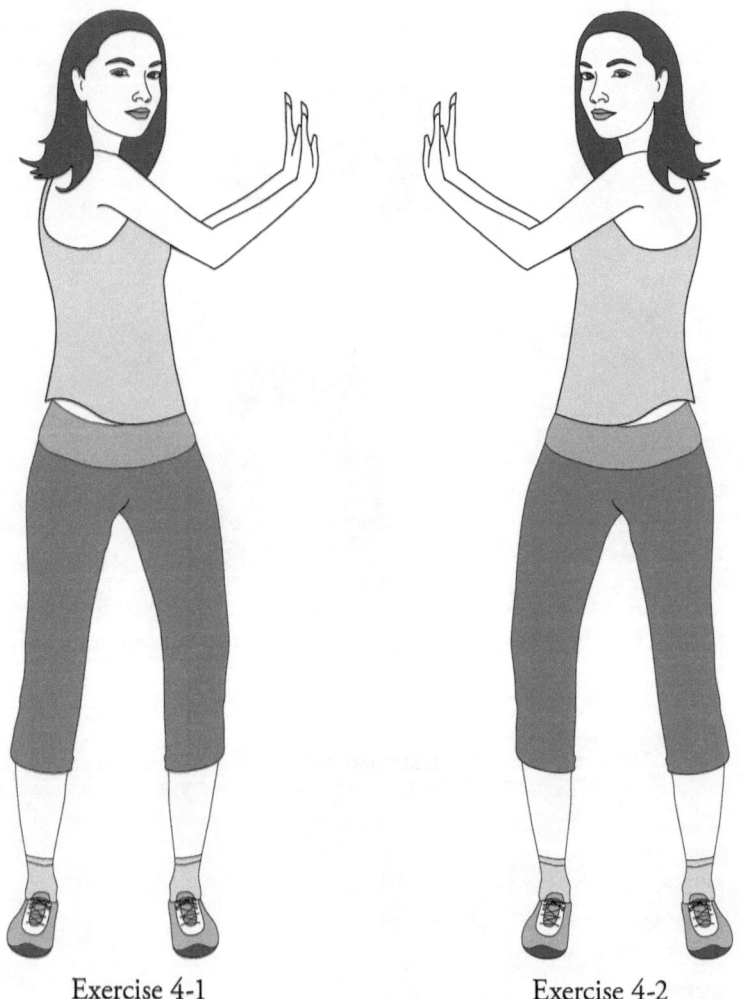

Exercise 4-1   Exercise 4-2

Exercise 5:

Perform a neck stretch in every direction (also rotation of the back). Hold for 30 seconds.

The fitness program

The fitness program should be repeated two to three times a week. It takes about eight to ten weeks for the muscles to be built so that the pain disappears.

Warm-up: 6-8 minutes

Back training: 20 minutes

Shoulders: 20 minutes

Neck: 10 minutes

Total: 1 hour

For your warm up, use the cross trainer or the bike.

Each exercise should be repeated for 2 to 3 sets, 10-15 repetitions per set.

Back

Exercise 1:

On the hyperextension bench, bend your spine forward and then come back to the starting position (see images below). Do the exercise with a straight back. If you have any questions on how to use the fitness equipment, please consult with a trainer in your fitness studio.

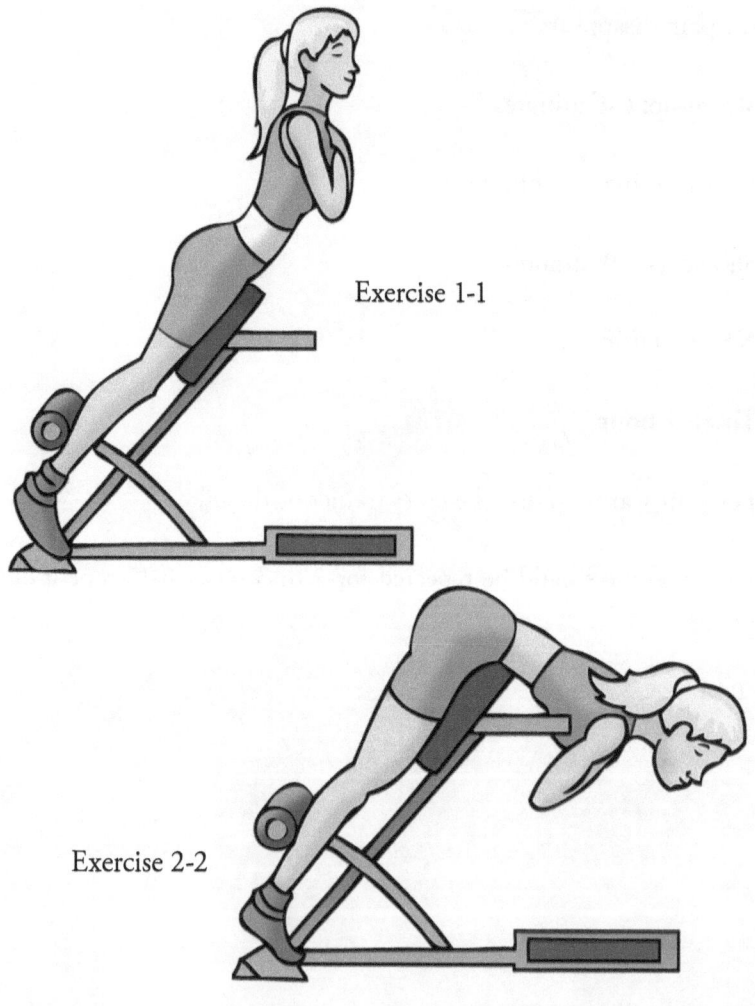

Exercise 1-1

Exercise 2-2

Exercise 2:

On the hyperextension bench, train the side stomach muscles by performing the bends sideways (see the image below). Repeat for 2-3 sets on the right and 2-3 sets on the left.

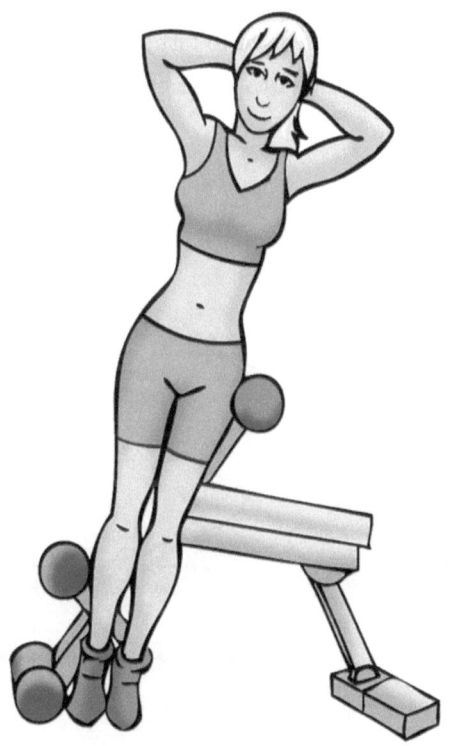

Exercise 2

Exercise 3:

Abdomen muscles

For this exercise, you need to use the cable and pulley machine in a seated position (see image below). Lie on your mat with stretched feet. Get up slowly for a sit up and bend towards your feet. It is important that you do this exercise <u>as slowly as possible</u> and with a little weight (start with 5 kilograms) for the machine. This movement might feel unnatural at first if you are used to fast sit ups. Think about twenty four mobile vertebrae on your spine as you perform the exercise.

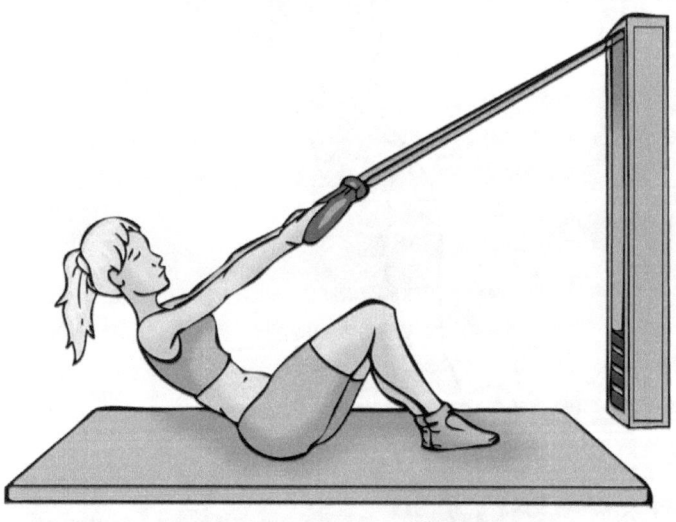

Exercise 3

Neck

Take a 1 kilogram weight. The head weighs approximately 6 kilograms, so the neck muscles also need to be trained to bend forward, backward, left, right, and rotate. Most of the time we only hold the head straight and this is why there is tension in the neck and shoulders building up.

For the rotation exercises, you will also need a rubber band.

Exercise 1: Bending the head forward

Lie down on a bench on your back. The head should be free to move. Hold the 1 kilogram weight with both hands and put it on the back of the head (see image). Repeat for 2 to 3 sets, 10-15 times per set. Use the full motion amplitude of the head.

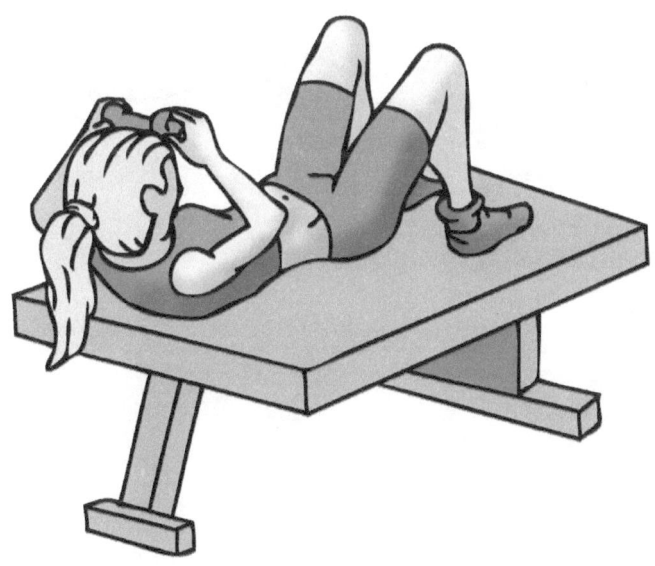

Exercise 1-1

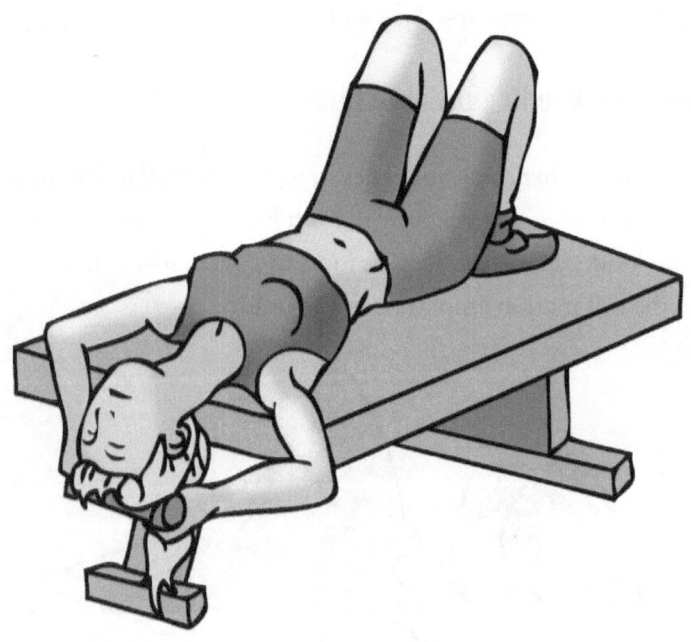

Exercise 1-2

Exercise 2: Bending the head backward

This exercise is the reverse of exercise 1. Now you lie down on your back and hold the weight with both hands on your forehead (see image below). Repeat for 2 to 3 sets, 10-15 times per set. Use the full motion amplitude of the head.

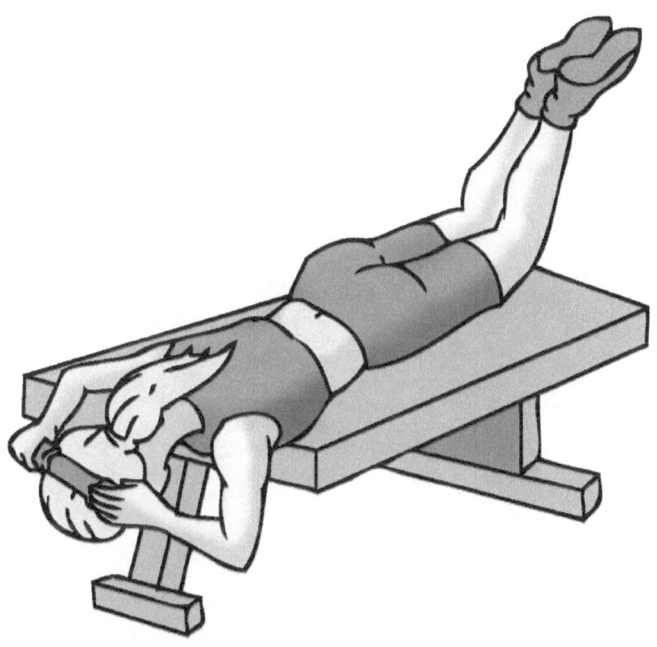

Exercise 2

Exercise 3: Bending the head sideways

Lie on your right side on the bench. Hold the 1 kg weight with your hand. Bend down and then up.

Now repeat on the left side.

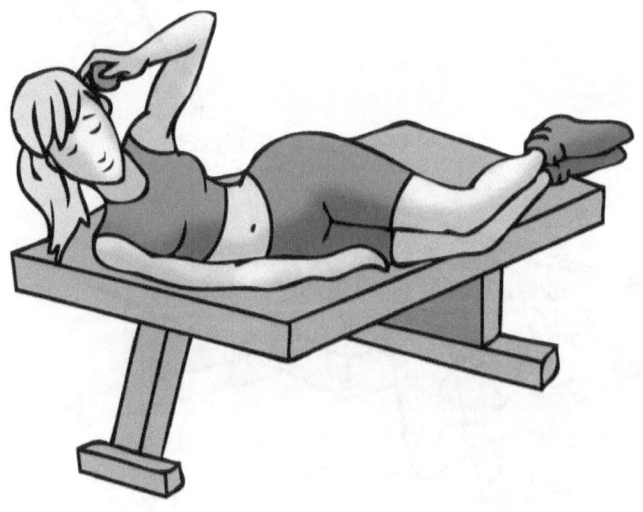

Exercise 3

Exercise 4: Rotation exercise with a rubber band

Wrap the rubber band around your forehead as shown in the picture. Perform a backwards rotation of the neck (trying to see behind your back).

Here, it is important that only the head turns (the upper body does not turn).

Think about moving a rope of pearls.

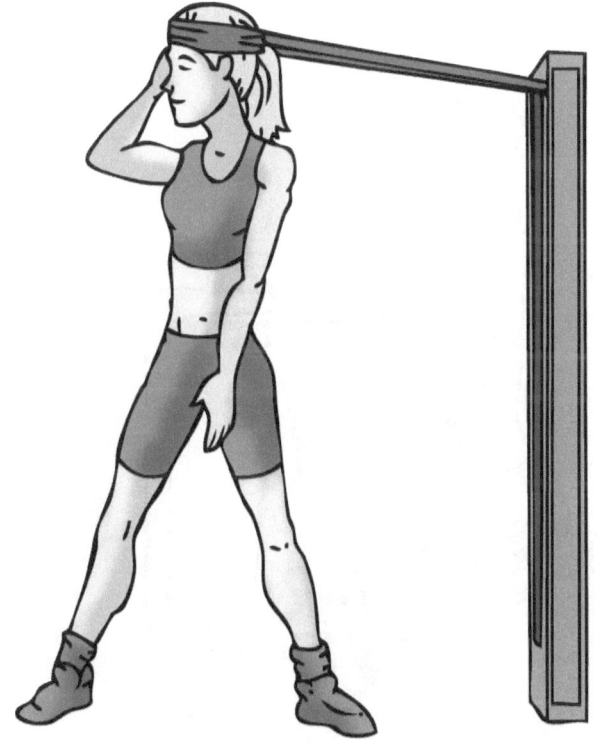

Exercise 4

Shoulder blades

It is important that the shoulder blades can move freely in all directions.

The suggested exercises help strengthen the muscles and practice the mobility.

<u>Exercise 1</u>: On the rower – pulling shoulder blades together

Normally, people are used to using the rower to train the arm. For the purposes of training the shoulder blades, pull only without bending the arms. You can imagine that you want to press the shoulder blades together.

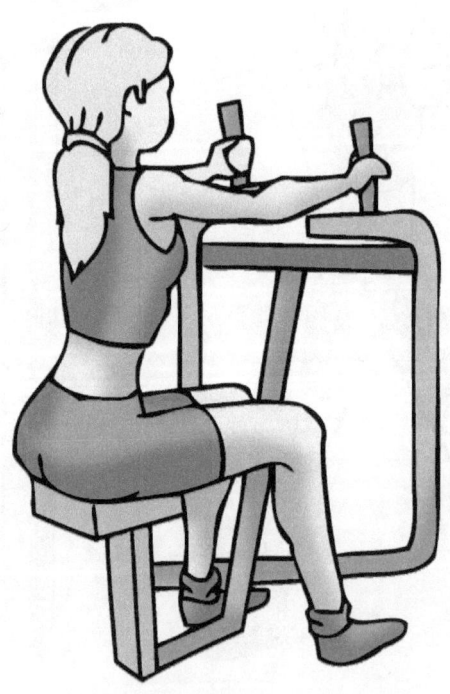

Exercise 2: Pulling shoulder blades to the ears with free weights

Take a weight in both hands (for example, try with 5 kilograms and adjust if necessary). With stretched arms, pull the shoulders towards the ears; hold the position for 3 seconds and release.

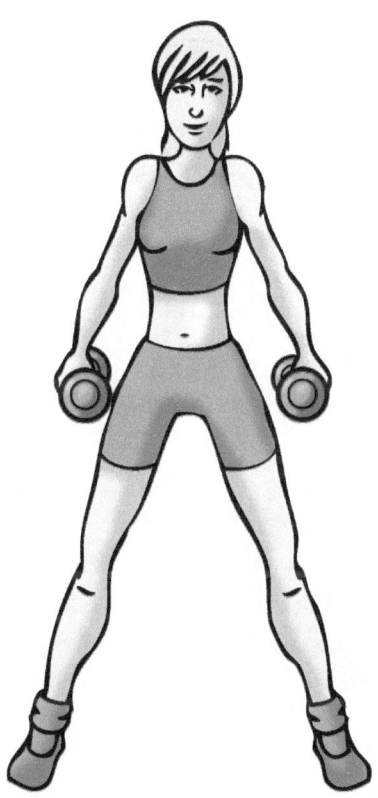

<u>Exercise 3</u>: On the triceps pusher, push the weight downward only from the shoulder blades (arms stay stretched).

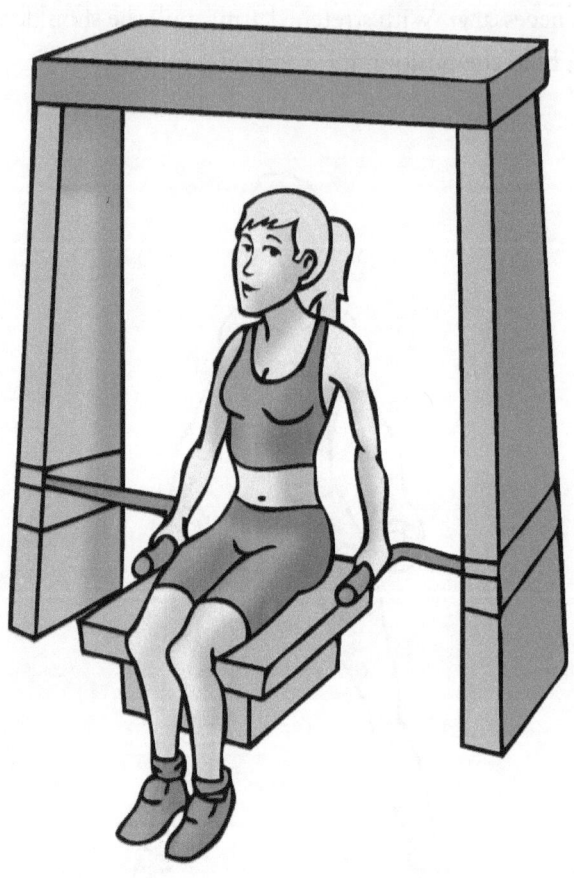

Exercise 4: Using the cable and pulley machine and sitting on your feet (see image below), train the shoulder blades by pulling the cable straight towards your body and releasing sideways.

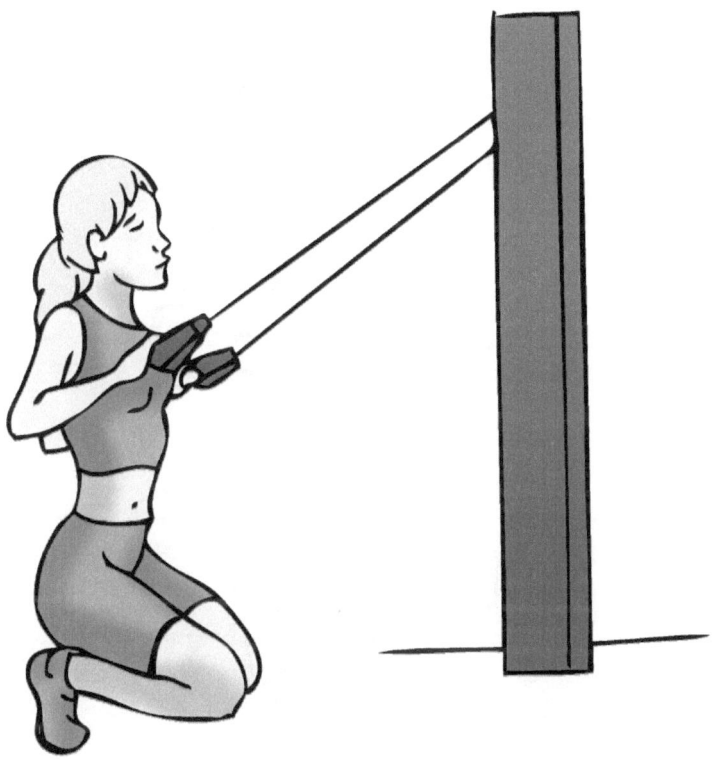

<u>Exercise 5</u>:

On the chest press, perform this exercise with stretched arms.

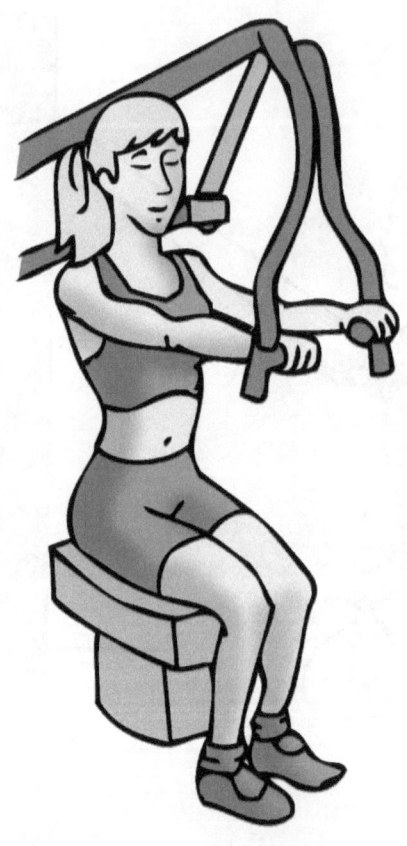

3.2. Healthy eating habits (and dieting)

When we discuss taking care of yourself and dealing with depression and burnout, developing healthy eating habits is a topic that deserves a chapter of its own. There are plenty of books written on this topic so if you have a deeper interest in learning about nutrition, check the references section for some tips of where to get started.

Most people are under time pressure during their short lunch breaks: they just grab a sandwich from a bakery and quickly eat it in front of the PC before continuing to sort through the hundreds of unimportant, unread e-mails.

People do not sit down to enjoy their coffee. Now we order "Coffee to go" in order to save time.

Eating, drinking, lunch breaks have become shorter and filled with pressure. No wonder that you are stressed out. Therefore, try to slow down – enjoy your lunch break and sit down for a coffee. Go for a ten minute walk after eating and consciously create the space and breaks you need in order to feel good at work.

As with everything else, "the healthy middle way" can be a good mantra for your choice of food. It is good to be aware of what is beneficial for your body and to treat your body like a good friend, giving it what it needs to stay functional. Most people have lost their feeling for food, so you first need to learn what is good for the body in order to make the best decisions for your nutrition.

Vitamin D and Omega 3 fat acids are very important for our nutrition. 95% of most Central Europeans have a lack of Vitamin D.

The macronutrients are proteins, carbohydrates and fats. In the industrial countries, more than 70% of our food is taken in the form of carbohydrates. People eat too much bread, sugar, noodles, rice and potatoes. However, should you decide you want to eat any of these, it is better to opt for rice or potatoes, which are high-quality carbohydrates.

The diet that most Western Europeans and Americans have leads to diabetes, obesity and the so-called metabolic syndrome. The metabolic syndrome is a modern age disease described as *"a disorder of energy utilization and storage, diagnosed by a co-occurrence of three out of five of the following medical conditions: abdominal (central) obesity, elevated blood pressure, elevated fasting plasma glucose, high serum triglycerides, and low high-density lipoprotein (HDL) levels."*[8]. Some of the important factors leading to it are stress, overweight and sedentary lifestyle (lack of movement). Being diagnosed with a metabolic syndrome increases the risk of cardiovascular disease and diabetes. Overeating, eating too many carbohydrates and eating under stress are the root causes for the above-mentioned diseases. It is therefore important that you spend time planning your nutrition and do not always rely on sandwiches and fast food offered by the bakery at the corner. Again, this does not mean to always control what you eat and to never allow yourself to eat some chocolate or ice-cream. **The "healthy middle way" should be your goal here as well.**

---

[8] *Wikipedia.* Wikimedia Foundation. Web. 27 Aug. 2015.

The more diverse your nutrition is, the better it is for your body. Here are some tips for you to keep in mind:

- Fish should often be part of your meal plan. Salmon, herring or sushi are a wonderful source of omega 3 fats.
- It is better to eat raw fruit rather than to order a freshly squeezed fruit juice. The juices contain mostly fibres and a lot of the nutritious ingredients have been squeezed away.
- A freshly squeezed juice will not satisfy your hunger.
- A salad with tuna fish or chicken is a very good choice for lunch.
- Try to reduce your intake of bread, sugar and noodles.
- For breakfast, you can prepare the following mix: 30% yoghurt, 70% curd cheese. Add sliced fruit and nuts. Instead of putting in ready-made cereal, add the following: oatmeal, chia seeds (1-2 soup spoons), and amaranth. You might have to order the amaranth and the chea seeds on-line or go to a bio supermarket, but this is worth the effort. One more tip: reduce the amount of cereal in your breakfast and increase the amount of curd cheese. Curd cheese contains protein.
- Have protein snacks ready to keep you going throughout your day. Cottage cheese and butter milk are great examples of such snacks.
- For salads and cooking, have these four sorts of oil ready: olive, rapeseed, pumpkin and linseed.
- Avoid sunflower oil and distilled oil.

Healthy eating and dieting

Every diet is stress for the body and muscles, and can lead to burnout if not done correctly.

Here are some tips related to dieting:

- Uncontrolled dieting is stress for the body and can lead to reduction of muscles as well as burnout.
- During your period of weight reduction, avoid juices, cola, cappuccino and alcohol. These contain "hidden" calories.
- For a week, write down everything that you consume. Having kept such a "diary" will help you become aware of which habits to change.
- You can calculate how much calories intake you need to keep your weight (without dieting). If you want to lose weight, subtract 500 calories from this number. You can either "lose" the calories from eating less or from adding more cardio exercises into your routine.

For example, a woman who weighs 52 kilograms and has an office job will have ca. 1800 calories available in order to keep her weight. She can eat more if she is willing to hit the gym for some cardio exercises a couple of times a week.

3.3. Other methods to support you:

<u>Shiatsu</u>

Shiatsu is an originally Japanese alternative medicine tradition which has become popular in the Western society in the last 30 years. A whole-body treatment lasts ca. one hour. Through a gentle touch and pressing with the thumbs, the Shiatsu practitioner helps you dissolve blockages in the body. The treatment reduces stress and supports change processes in your life. It is recommended to book a couple of sessions in order to experience the best effects (but, of course, it is your call what you want to do ☺).

Shiatsu supports the self-healing power of the body and gives you extra energy to implement the decisions you make to change your life. The Shiatsu Society in Germany has its own Web-page listing all certified practitioners in order to avoid fraud. Check whether there is a similar organized agency in your country. As I already mentioned before, it is worth spending some time researching and asking questions before and when try anything new, in order to figure out whether this treatment is something for you.

Qi Gong

Qi Gong is a branch of the traditional Chinese medicine. During the Qi Gong practice, you learn to consciously perceive the Qi, which in Chinese means "life energy".

With smooth movements, the Qi is passed in the imagination to the parts of the body that need it. This activity helps release muscle tension. The person comes to rest, becomes more flexible and more relaxed. Qi Gong also increases sleep quality.

Tai Qi

Tai Qi is a type of martial art (shadow boxing) which belongs to the Chinese cultural heritage. The person is practicing action and reaction images with wave-like slow movements in order to ward off an imaginary opponent. It is also possible to practice Tai Qi in a seated position.

Because of its unusual slowness, Tai Qi trains the smallest muscles as well. This art of training increases flexibility, reduces back pain, strengthens the body and boosts the inner balance. Tai Qi leads to relaxation and a deepened concentration.

Yoga

Yoga is one of the philosophical schools in India. According to the teacher Patanjali, yoga is a way of following certain rules, similar to the Christian commandments.

The training positions show your personal boundaries. At the same time, you concentrate on the present moment. This combination makes you more flexible, also in the way of thinking. Yoga can minimize back pain, depressive symptoms, and stress. It is important to consult a doctor if you are not sure whether you are allowed to perform all motions, because in some cases, bending the back can be harmful.

4. Self-forgiveness

Stress and burnout have manifested in your life to show you that you have not been taking proper care of yourself. Since you are now reading this book, you have already made the first step towards changing your situation. You should be proud of yourself and take it easy.

Self-forgiveness is a process, and it might take some time for your mind to adjust. As with any new habit, practice taking care of yourself and checking in with your body about its needs on a daily basis. Do your meditation practice and physical exercises regularly. Learn to say no when your boundaries have been crossed.

With all of your new habits in place, it will be easier for you to accept and forgive yourself.

Most people are harsher in judging themselves than anyone else. Observe your self-talk. How often do you say to yourself: "I am such an idiot", "I am not smart enough", "I will never be able to figure this out"? Now transform these sentences into positives: "I still do not know this, but I will figure it out", "With patience, I have the capacity to acquire this new skill", "I am capable if I put my mind to it". How do these new sentences feel?

It is important that you focus on the positives in your life and create positive self-affirmations. Be gentle to yourself and remind yourself often that you are doing your best and are in the process of developing new habits.

You may be harsh on yourself because of the way situations evolved differently from what you expected in your professional or private life. When you are experiencing the pain and the mess of everything seemingly going wrong, you keep reliving the past and asking yourself what you could have done better. Stop this behaviour.

In such moments, it is even more important to see the positive sides of the situations and to look for what lessons you learnt from them, and how this experience can make you a better person. For example, if a relationship fell apart or a job was not the right fit for you, you can analyze what you can do differently next time. Do this with compassion and treat yourself like a child learning to walk. Parents do not scold their children for falling down when they still learn how to walk. So, why would you want to punish yourself for your mistakes given that you did your best at that particular moment?

5. Self-acceptance

If you are at a point in your life where you have been through some tough experiences, you might blame yourself for what is happening. Be nice to yourself. It is very easy to fall in the trap of focusing only on the negative feelings and emotions. You might also be someone who does not share these feelings for the fear of not being accepted or feeling ridiculous, which makes it even more difficult for you to process your emotions and can lead to depression.

There is a nice exercise which can help you focus on your positive qualities[9]. The exercise is called the "self-worth" pot. Take an A4 piece of paper and draw a pot like the one below. Draw a line approximately in the middle. Above the line, write down your qualities and experiences which enhance your self-worth. Below the line, write down the activities which deplete you. Tape this sheet on your drawer and continue filling it in on a regular basis. You will be surprised about how much you have to offer to the world and just do not think about.

---

[9] This exercise has been shared with me by Carsten Stepan.

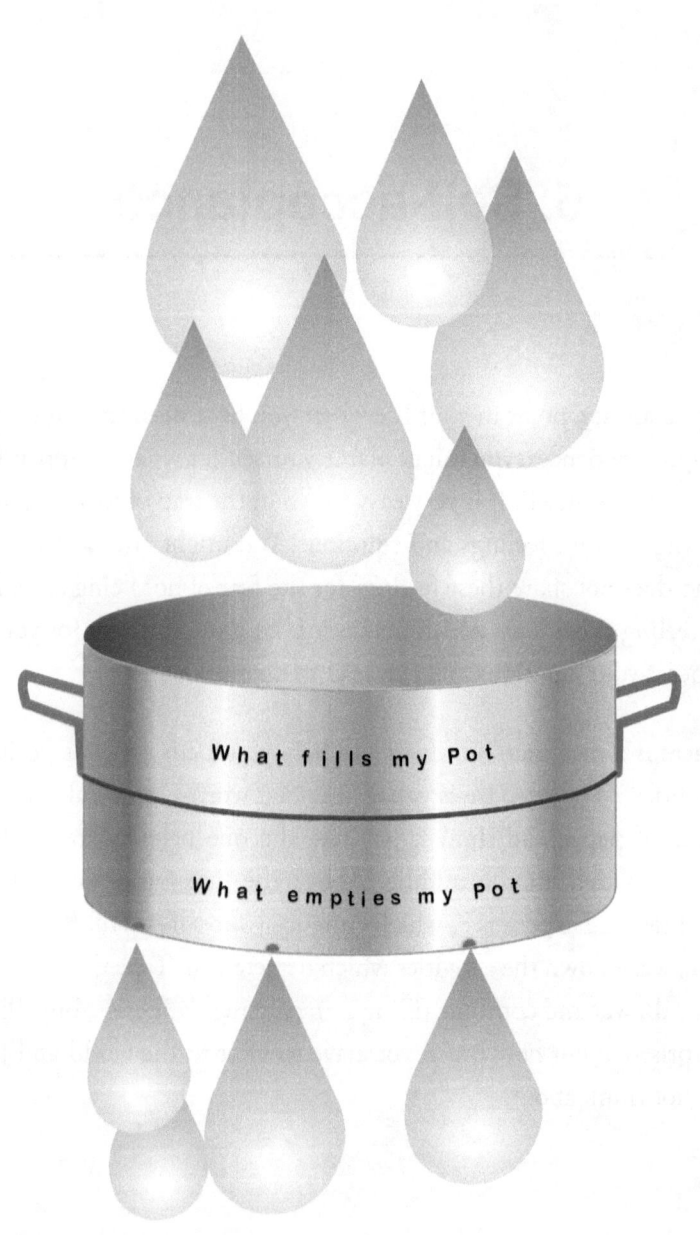

What fills my Pot

What empties my Pot

For example, this is how part of my "self-worth pot" looks like:

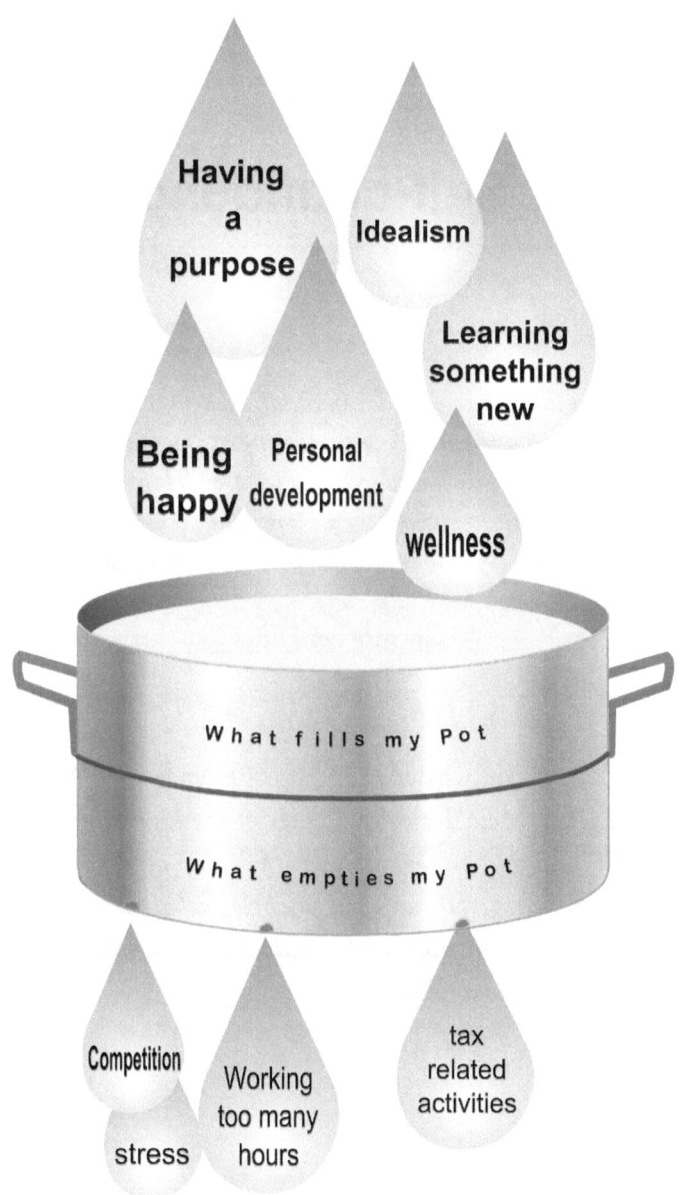

Now, it's your turn…

6. Self-confidence

----

*"First and foremost, if we maintain healthy emotional
boundaries and direct love and kindness inwards, we are
taking care of ourselves and secondly we are giving a subliminal
message to others about how we wish to be treated. People
tend to subconsciously treat us how we treat ourselves."*

— Christopher Dines —

Stress can significantly reduce our self-confidence level. As the The
Counseling and Mental Health Center of the University of Texas
defines: *"Too much stress can seriously affect your physical and mental
well-being. Recurrent physical and psychological stress can diminish
self-esteem, decrease interpersonal effectiveness, and create a cycle of
self-blame and self-doubt."*[10]

-----

[10] "Managing Stress." Stress. Web. 28 Aug. 2015.

Below is a list of positive affirmations that you can print out and refer to if you feel that negativity habits come back to your life[11]:

CHALLENGES HELP ME GROW

I CAN SEE STRESSFUL SITUATIONS AS CHALLENGES

CHALLENGES BRING ME OPPORTUNITIES

I CAN CHOOSE A POSITIVE FRAME OF MIND

I CAN HANDLE WHATEVER COMES

I CAN STAY CALM UNDER PRESSURE

A lot of women define self-worth based on looks. Of course, it is important that you take care of yourself and your wardrobe in order to feel good in your own skin. However, I find it sad that so many women base their self-worth on comparisons to model images flashing at us from glossy magazines. The moment you start comparing yourself to others, you will always find people who are younger or better looking than you are. I would encourage you to look deeper instead. What else do you have to offer to the world? How do you make a difference in the lives of the people around you? How can you be a good friend and listener?

In addition, self-confidence comes from living an authentic life and speaking your truth. Voicing your truth can be scary at first. It is best to start with situations in which the outcome is not very important. Once you voice your opinion, be prepared to defend your point of view and not always give in. Stress and a lack of self-worth

---

[11] Scott, M.S. "Positive Affirmations for Stress Relief." Web. 28 Aug. 2015.

result from doing things we disagree with. Have the courage to say no if you are asked to stay in the office after office hours. Have the courage to set a boundary with a family member if they have behaved in a disrespectful manner. The action of standing up for yourself is very empowering and gives you the courage to believe in yourself and your capabilities.

If you have a void to fill – if you need a larger support network, then go out and explore new areas of interest. You can make a list of the things that you have wanted to try but postponed because of taking care of the priorities of other people. Then, step out of your comfort zone and do these activities. Breaking away from your daily routine and proving to yourself that you can take on a challenge will help you develop better self-confidence.

Sometimes you will have to be your own cheerleader along the way. When someone tries to put you down, choose to stand up for yourself. You can try this when you have a salary negotiation or when you set up the rules for a relationship. Try this new behavior until it starts to feel natural. Acting with authenticity and standing up for yourself even in difficult life situations can be a great boost for your self-confidence.

Think of your own needs and put yourself first in relationships. By putting yourself and your happiness first, you teach people to respect you. The ones in your life who cannot accept your new-found self-confidence will disappear. You will then be able to draw in people to yourself who truly appreciate you for who you are.

7. Live! Redefine your life

Redefining your life does not always have to be drastic (at least not everything at once). Of course, you may come to the realization that you do want to totally change your life direction and try out something completely new – travel the world, open a small coffee place or turn your hobby into an on-line business.

However, this does not always need to be the case. A lot of people like what they are doing and you might just need to change your daily tasks or switch departments in order to find the workplace where you feel valued and appreciated.[12] There is even a process called "job crafting" which can help shift the focus of your everyday work without necessarily needing to switch departments or companies:

"The Job Crafting™ Exercise helps you make your job more engaging and fulfilling. This interactive tool allows you to view your job as a flexible set of building blocks. Using this unique perspective, you create a visual plan for redesigning your job to better suit your values, strengths, and passions. The result is a more optimal fit between you and your job, boosting your happiness and effectiveness at work."[13]

---

[12] "Unhappy at Work? Try Hacking Your Job." WSJ. Web. 26 Aug. 2015.
[13] "Job Crafting Store." Job Crafting LLC. Web. 28 Aug. 2015.

If you are interested in the job crafting exercise, check out the booklet which you can get from the following Web-site: http:// jobcrafting.com/

If you decide to apply for a new job, take some time to write down what the "must haves" are in this job. For example, you might find it important to have security, team work and no overtime hours. Think about whether you would be willing to accept a lower pay check or more routine tasks in return.

Take the time to check out the reviews of previous and current employees of the firm that you are applying to. There will be plenty of information on bigger firms available on the Internet. If you can, talk to employees and ask about their experiences with the firm. You can use career networking Web-Sites such as XING and LINKED IN for this purpose. Do not shy away to mention at your interview that work-life balance is important for you and ask how this topic is handled in the company. Check out the Company's Web-site and see whether they "advertise themselves" as an employee-friendly company. See whether you will have access to a gym and other perks that will make your work life easier.

If you decide that you want to change the relationship dynamics in your current relationship, be bold enough and state your needs. You must have the confidence to speak up your truth in an authentic way; otherwise the people around you (in particular, your partner/ spouse) might not be aware of having hurt you.

If you want to find a new partner, first take the time to write and analyze what qualities you are looking for in this partner. Be brutally honest in writing down your needs so that you can compare them with the character traits of the people you meet. Trying to fit in a lifestyle which you do not enjoy and having your basic needs not met can be a source of deep frustration and dissatisfaction. Therefore, choose carefully.

It is important that you listen to your inner voice which you have hopefully developed by now following the methodology outlined in this book.

HAVE A GREAT LIFE! BE AUTHENTIC AND STEP UP FOR YOURSELF! THE BETTER YOU KNOW YOURSELF, THE MORE YOU WILL SHOW UP FOR YOUR LIFE.

GOOD LUCK!

Space for your own notes

8. References and addresses for more information

Carsten Stepan

A center for body feeling and awareness

http://www.pure-bewusstleben.de

Qi Gong and Tai Chi – the Shaolin way

http://www.shaolin-quan.de/

Shiatsu Germany

Eimsbütteler Str. 53-55

22769 Hamburg

Tel. 0049 – 40 – 85506736

info@shiatsu-gsd.de

www.shiatsu-gsd.de

Rosanna Capelli

Shiatsu practitioner

Meetpoint Health

Helene-Mayer-Ring 10

Munich, Germany

Tel. 0049 89 15883637

Ale Cantu

Consciousness Coaching

info@alecantu.com

http://alecantu.com

The Job Crafting Exercise

"Job Crafting Store." *Job Crafting LLC*. Web. 28 Aug. 2015.

http://jobcrafting.com/

Bibliography

"Festhalten - Loslassen - Festhalten - Loslassen." *Philosophisch Leben*. 17 Feb. 2014. Web. 26 Aug. 2015.

https://philosophischleben.wordpress.com/2014/02/17/festhalten-loslassen-festhalten-loslassen/

"Managing Stress." Stress. Web. 28 Aug. 2015.

http://cmhc.utexas.edu/stress.html

"Thich-nhat-hanh-quotes." - *Mystical Earth Adventures*™. Web. 26 Aug. 2015.

http://www.mysticalearthadventures.com/thich-nhat-hanh-quotes.html

Scott, M.S. "Positive Affirmations for Stress Relief." Web. 28 Aug. 2015. http://stress.about.com/od/optimismspirituality/a/freeaffirmation.htm

Tornambe, M.D. "Does Stress Make You Ugly?" *The Huffington Post*. TheHuffingtonPost.com. Web. 26 Aug. 2015.

"Unhappy at Work? Try Hacking Your Job." WSJ. Web. 26 Aug. 2015.

http://www.wsj.com/articles/unhappy-at-work-try-hacking-your-job-1439313771

What Is Qigong?" *Energy Arts*. Web. 27 Aug. 2015. http://www.energyarts.com/what-qigong

"What Does It Mean To Be Centered?" *What Does It Mean To Be Centered?* Web. 27 Aug. 2015.

https://www.jiyushinkai.org/centered.html

"Why Some Women Are Burning Out in Their 20's and 30's."
Psychology Today. Web. 26 Aug. 2015.

https://www.psychologytoday.com/blog/pressure-proof/201411/
why-some-women-are-burning-out-in-their-20s-and-30s

Davis, William. *Weizenwampe: Warum Weizen Dick Und Krank Macht*. München: Goldmann, 2013. Print.

Enders, Giulia. *Darm Mit Charme*. Berlin: Ullstein Buchverlage, 2014. Print.

Gonder, Ulrike, and Nicolai Worm. *Mehr Fett! Warum Wir Mehr Fett Brauchen, Um Gesund Und Schlank Zu Sein ; Liebeserklärung an Einen Zu Unrecht Verteufelten Nährstoff*. Lünen: Systemed, 2010. Print.

Worm, Nicolai. *Heilkraft D*. Lünen: Systemed-Verl., 2009. Print.